YOGA

The Best Yoga Top Yoga Poses to Relieve Stress and Gain Strength

WHITLEY SMITH

TABLE OF CONTENT

INTRODUCTION

Yoga is a traditional kind of physical activity that emphasizes breathing, flexibility, and strength to improve mental and physical well-being. Yoga began in India approximately five thousand years ago and has been adopted in other nations in several different forms. The two primary parts of yoga are breathing and posture. Yoga postures are a series of moving activities meant to elevate flexibility and strength.

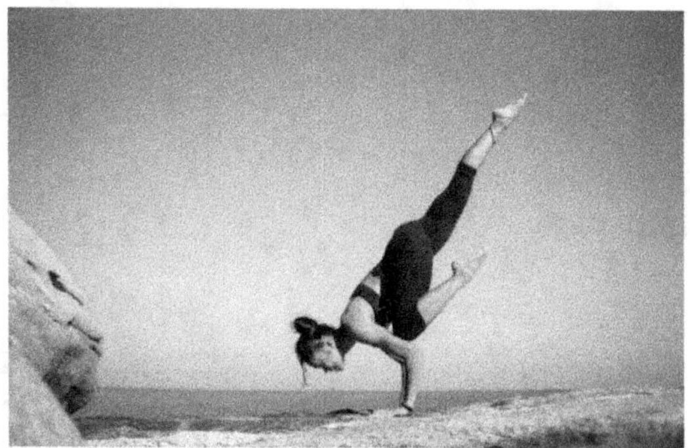

HEALTH BENEFIT OF YOGA

Yoga has a lot of advantages and is enjoyable to practice.

Yoga is sometimes likened to naturopathy due to its curative

qualities and the benefits it offers to physical and mental

health. You may enhance your overall health real quick by

practicing yoga, which is both natural and entirely free.

To be in good health involves more than just taking care of

yourself; it also involves associating yourself with positive

thoughts.

Regular practice of yoga:

    i.   minimizes anxiety

    ii.   aids digestion

iii.   enhances balance

iv.   eases menstrual discomfort

v.   minimizes headache and fatigue

vi.   aids asthma

vii.   soothes symptoms of menopause.

Let's group the benefits of yoga into two which are:

i.   **Physical benefit**

ii.   **Mental benefit**

Physical Benefits

✓ Yoga poses to aid in softly toning up the range of motion in the body muscles and joints.

✓ Yoga when done with breathing exercises helps in blood circulation and heart improvement.

✓ Yoga poses enhance body balance and stability in order to prevent falling.

✓ Pranayama for instance helps to maintain a stable healthy lifestyle which in turn enhances respiration.

✓ 5Yoga is a great exercise to get rid of excessive fat in the body. So, if you want to lose weight, yoga is your go-to workout.

✓ Regular practice of yoga helps one to be more active in other sporting activities.

✓ Yoga exercises provide resistance through the body weight for the muscles to be stretched and strengthened.

Mental Benefits

✓ Stress relief is one of the most appreciative mental benefits of yoga. This is so because yoga comprises both relaxation methods and physical activities.

✓ Yoga aids in keeping your mind at ease and also makes you concentrate a great deal. It is hard to lose focus after a session of yoga

✓ Yoga enhances the rate of individual self-awareness. It makes you know and appreciate yourself more.

✓ With the constant practice of yoga, depression has no
way in your life. The practice of yoga automatically
lifts your spirit and boosts your self-confidence in
that there is no room for anxiety.

✓ Yoga helps you live in the moment. You enjoy every
moment more as you practice yoga and with time you
leave the past and stop worrying about the future.

✓ The amount of self-worth yoga practice brings to one
is second to none. You see yourself being confident
in yourself every time.

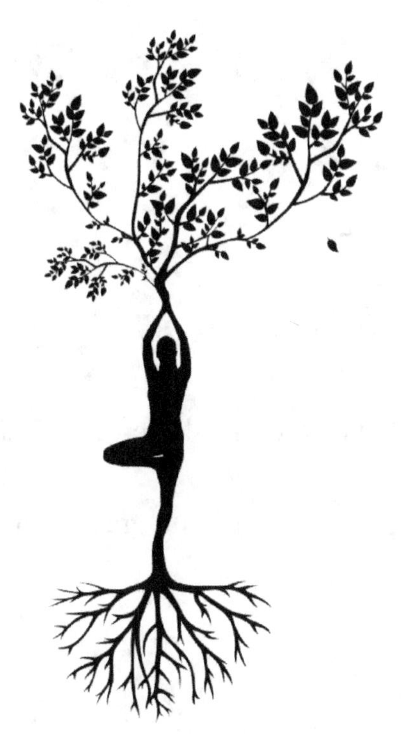

YOGA POSES

Mountain Pose (Tadasana)

Category: Beginner

The Mountain Pose is typically **starting posture for all standing yoga poses**. It is also occasionally referred to as **the resting position** and is a great position for improving posture.

Directions

- ✓ Begin by standing with your feet close to each other so your big toes meet, but with your heels moderately separated.

- ✓ As necessary, move back and forth or side to side so your weight is uniformly spread over your feet.

- ✓ YYourpalms should be facing forward in an open-handed gesture as you relax your arms.

- ✓ Assume a rope pushing you into a straight line by passing up through your feet and the back of your skull.

- ✓ As your tailbone pulls down toward the floor, pull your shoulder blades back towards each other.

- ✓ Maintain the position for one-minute while breathing smoothly.

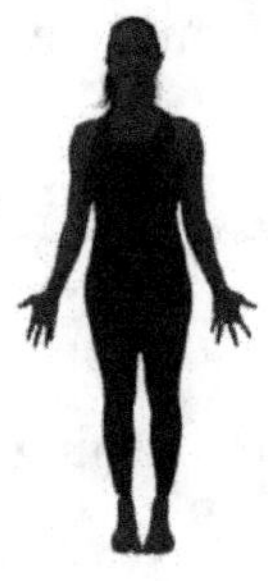

Standing Forward Bend

Category: Beginner

While tightening the muscles and loosening the hamstrings and calves, this pose can also activate the kidneys and the liver, which could aid in better digestion.

Directions

- ✓ Release your body forward on an exhalation, bending downward.

- ✓ If your back is under too much strain, flex your knees

- ✓ Don't push your body forward; rather, curl your hands over your heels. Your head should drop loosely from your spine when you relax your neck.

- ✓ Maintain your posture for ten to thirty seconds before rising to your feet or bending forward at the waist while you breathe in.

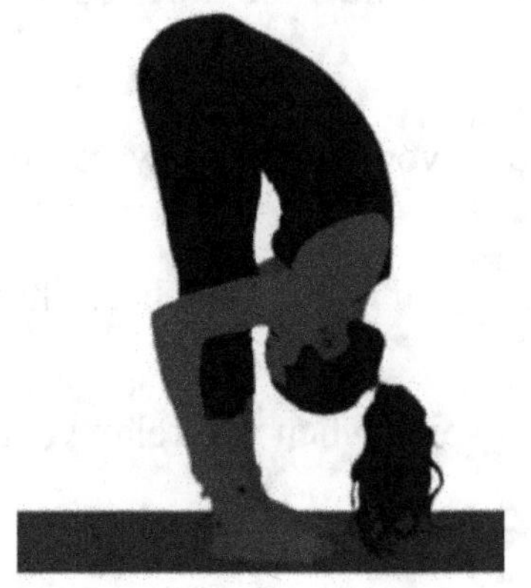

Palm Tree Pose

Category: Beginner

The Palm Tree Pose, also **known as the Upward Salute**, is one of the most fundamental poses in yoga and is **appropriate for beginners**. It is frequently used as a warm-up to reduce tension before transitioning into a more rigorous yoga asana.

Directions

- ✓ Begin in Mountain Pose.

- ✓ Extend your arms as high as possible in the sky, extending your spine and letting an unseen rope raise you onto your toes.

- ✓ Put your hands together behind your head and breathe in.

- ✓ Return to standing level on your feet and breathe out as you go farther to the right.

- ✓ As you breathe in, pause for a second and then return to the center.

- ✓ Redo the center stretch, then switch to the right side.

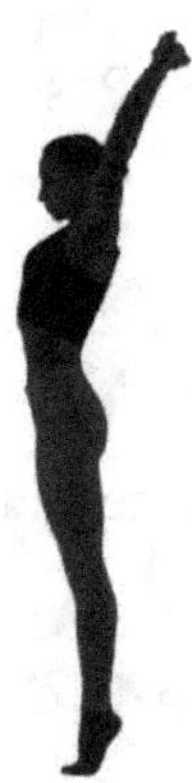

Downward-facing Dog Pose

Category: Beginner

One of the most popular yoga asanas is downward-facing dog pose, and for valid cause. It is an immensely useful pose that offers an all-over stretch. It also provides an outstanding changeover between standing positions and floor positions.

Directions

- ✓ Start on your hands and knees on the ground, with your knees just underneath your hips and your hands just in front of your shoulders.

- ✓ Breathe out and raise your knees off the ground. Do not lock your knees; instead, slowly extend both legs.

✓ Keep your entire body extended rather than moving your feet in the direction of your hands. Maintain this position for thirty seconds.

✓ To unwind, softly flex your knees as you breathe out and come back to your hands and knees, bring your hands forward into a plank position, or slide one foot forward into a lunge position.

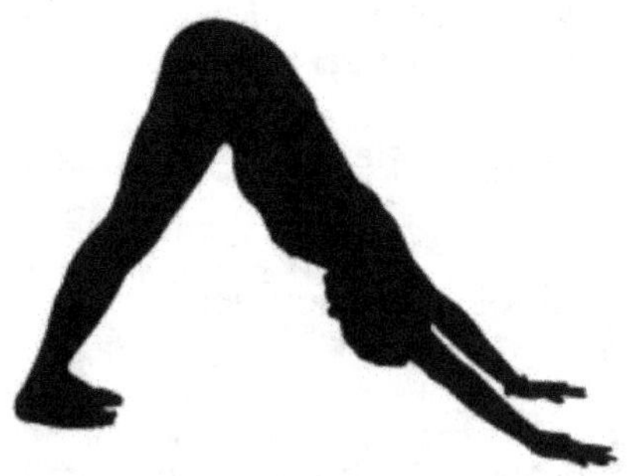

High Lunge

Category: Beginner

High lunge aids in lower body strengthening, expand the chest, and improves balance and flexibility for starters. It also acts as a foundation for tougher poses.

Directions

- ✓ Start with the downward-facing dog position, raise one of your back feet and advance it to settle between your hands.

- ✓ Put your hands on the ground by your feet while in a half-standing forward bend, then stretch one foot backward.

- ✓ Make your weight level to the ground while lowering your front knee over the heel to make your spine square to the ground.

- ✓ Place your weight in the center of your feet and elevate your torso till it's straight.

- ✓ Inhale while stretching your arms far into the air toward the sky.

- ✓ Maintain the position while breathing properly for ten to thirty seconds. With every breath, you take in, expand your torso while maintaining an unobstructed forward gaze.

✓ Put your hands outside of your front feet to exit the
posture, then either move your back leg forward to
return to the downward-facing dog or move your
front leg backward to do so.

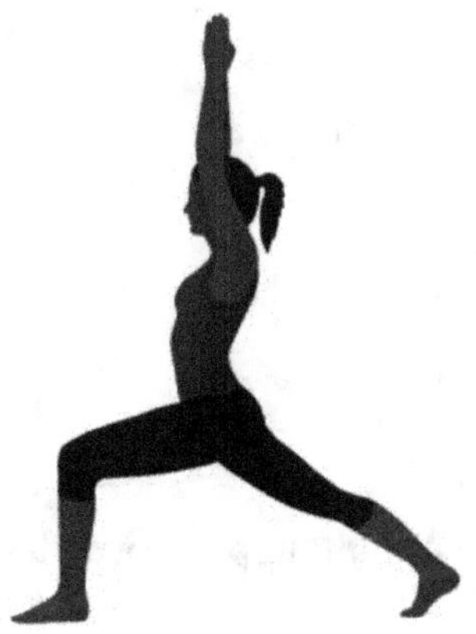

Chair Pose

Category: Beginner

Chair Pose helps strengthens thighs and ankles, while toning

shoulders, butt, hips, and back. Also

stimulates the heart and diaphragm.

Directions

✓ Begin in the mountain pose or tadasana.

✓ Lift your arms level to the ground as you breathe in, palms facing inside.

- ✓ Breathe out and bend your knees so that you appear to be sitting down in a chair till your spine forms the proper angle with your thighs.

- ✓ Maintain your inner thighs parallel to each other and press to the back with your shoulder blades as though you were resisting on the seat of a chair.

- ✓ Raise your arms above your head and maintain that position between thirty and sixty seconds.

- ✓ Breathe in while bending your knees to exit this position.

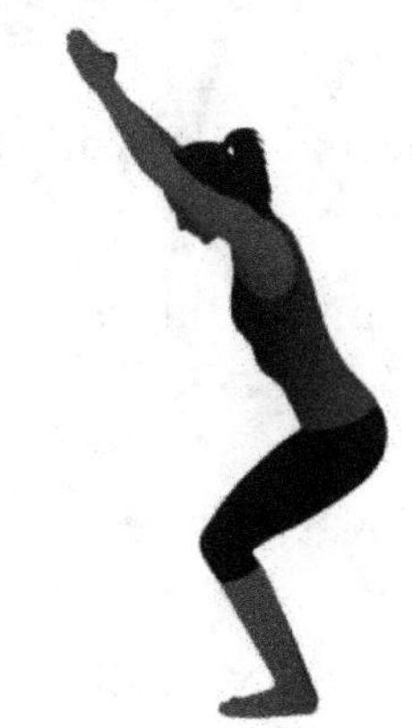

Triangle Pose

Category: Beginner

One of the most fundamental yoga poses, the triangle pose has many variations. The triangle Pose improves the core while stretching the ankles, legs, thighs, and feet.

Moreover, it stretches the hips, calf muscles, spine, hamstrings, and hip joints while also enhancing balance and exposing the chest to aid in better breathing.

Directions

✓ To begin, stand on your exercise mat with your legs wide open wide (roughly three to four feet apart) and your toes pointed front.

- ✓ The right foot should be turned 90 degrees out, and the left foot should be turned in around 45 degrees.

- ✓ Raise your hands to your hips and turn your hips so you are now facing the mat's end.

- ✓ Breathing out, bow at the hips and tilt your head to the right till it's level with the ground.

- ✓ Expand the spine while maintaining your left hand on your hips, then drop your right hand to the ground just behind your right foot.

- ✓ Lift your left arm upward as you breathe in.

✓ Breathe out deeply and lift your gaze up at your top hand

✓ Maintain the position between ten and thirty seconds, then lower your left hand and return to the center.

✓ Switch sides and repeat the process.

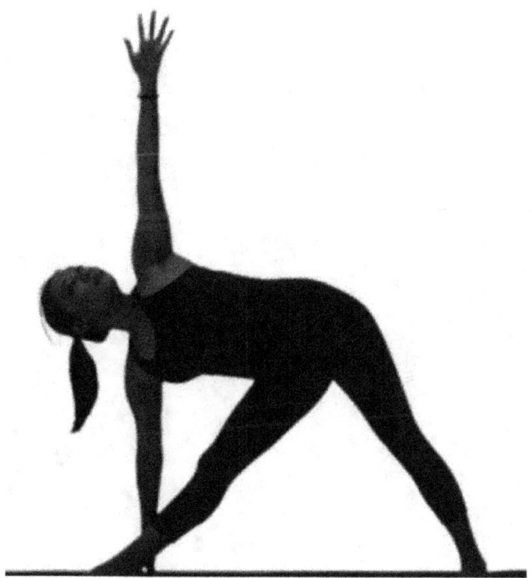

Staff Pose

Category: Beginner

Another of the most essential yoga poses that can be used as a link while going between one pose and another is the staff pose. It also **offers complete body strengthening and improves general flexibility.**

Directions

- ✓ Begin by sitting down and extending your legs straight out in front of you.

- ✓ Put your palms down on the floor to either side of you.

✓ Feel a cord tugging up on your spine and a second dragging you forward from your heels.

✓ Your feet should be stretched with your toes facing up.

✓ Deeply breathe in and gradually breathe out while maintaining your body upright and your spine balanced.

✓ Retain for between thirty and sixty seconds.

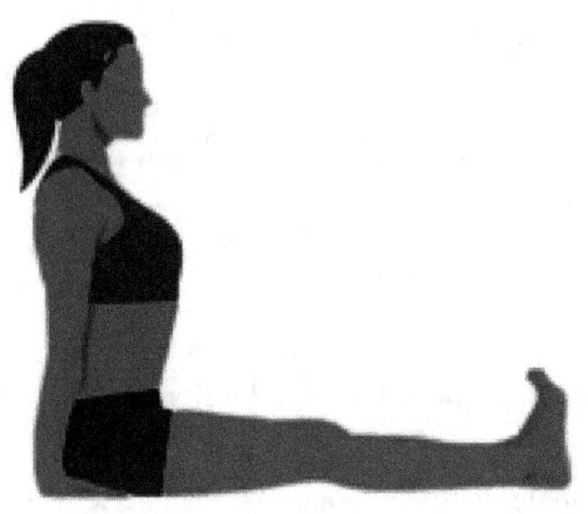

Easy Pose

Category: Beginner

Easy Pose helps **straighten out the hips and stretches the spine**. It also improves inner calmness and stretches the backbone. This yoga pose is beginners worthy.

Directions

- ✓ Begin this yoga in the in staff pose.

- ✓ Bring your left leg in so your left foot is below your right thigh.

- ✓ Draw your right leg in till it sits beneath your left hip. Inhale, lengthen your spine, and rise as high as you can.

- ✓ Hold the position for a few seconds while breathing softly.

- ✓ Untwist your legs, then switch to the other side.

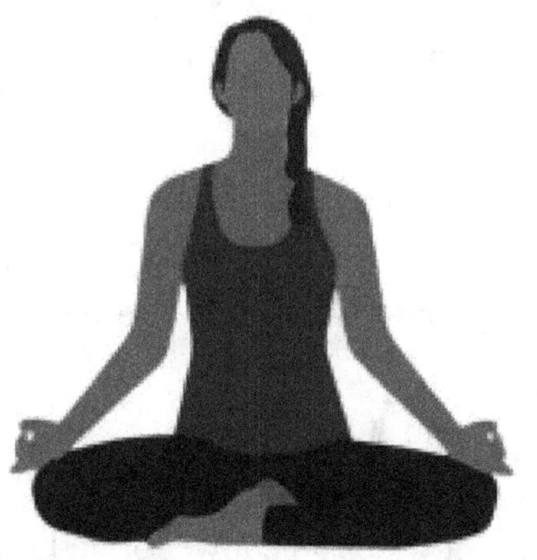

Bound Ankle Pose

Category: Beginner

The bound angle pose assists in **enhancing flexibility in the back, inner thigh, and knee**. It is also helpful for **easing period pain and can help pregnant women birth more easily**. Moreover, it widens the lower back, hips, and chest. Because **this is how cobblers often sit** while at work, it is occasionally referred to as the **Cobbler's Pose.**

Directions

- ✓ To begin, straighten your spine while sitting on the ground.

- ✓ Bring your feet as close or as contact as practicable while folding your knees.

- ✓ Your legs should have the appearance of butterfly wings as much as feasible.

- ✓ Wrap your fingers around your toes. Holding your feet firmly in place with your hands while pulling your torso forth with your back level and your chest open.

- ✓ Gently breathe in and pull your knees and hips into the ground with your elbows. Maintain this stance for twenty seconds.

- ✓ Breathe out, loosen your thighs then return to the upright position.

- ✓ Redo the process till you feel at ease and loosen.

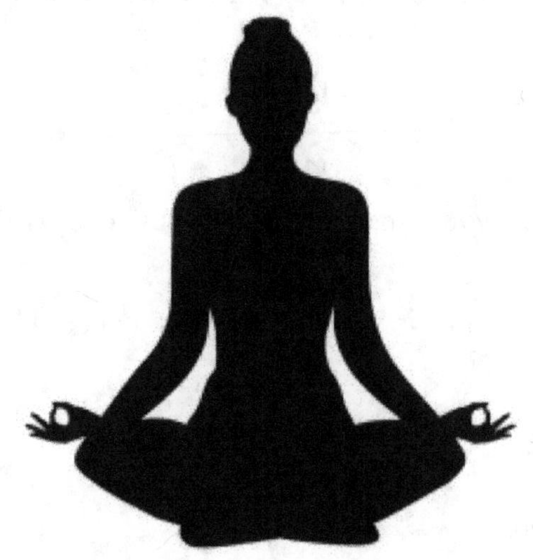

Half Lord of the Fishes Pose

Category: Beginner

The Half Lord of the Fishes Pose extends the shoulders, hips,

and back. It also

enhances blood circulation, improves abdomen, and braces

obliques.

Directions

- ✓ While on the floor, begin this yoga in a Staff Pose.

- ✓ Interwine your right foot over the outside of the left

  thigh, curving your knee so it points towards the sky.

- ✓ Curve your left knee to move your left foot under

  your right buttock.

✓ Curve your left arm upward and put your left elbow outside of your right knee and put your right hand on the ground behind you.

✓ Spin as far to the right as you can, while maintaining both buttocks on the ground.

✓ Maintain this position for one minute, breathing softly and turning slightly with each exhalation.

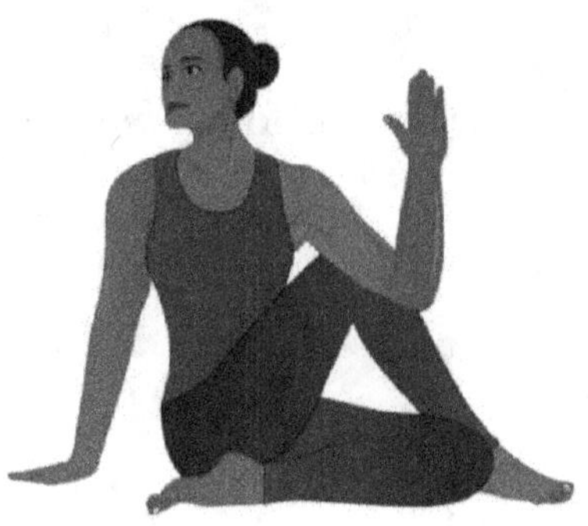

Table Pose

Category: Beginner

From the Table Pose, you can change into a variety of other positions, such as the Cow/Cat or Balanced Table Pose. Also, it improves lung capacity by strengthening the hands, arms, and shoulders, stretching the spine, toning the back muscles, and expanding the chest.

Directions

- ✓ To start, kneel on all fours, with your hands under your shoulders and your knees aligned beneath your hips.

- ✓ Maintain a flat back, with your head, neck, and back aligned with your spine.

- ✓ Your back should be totally straight from the back of your skull to the apex of your tailbone.

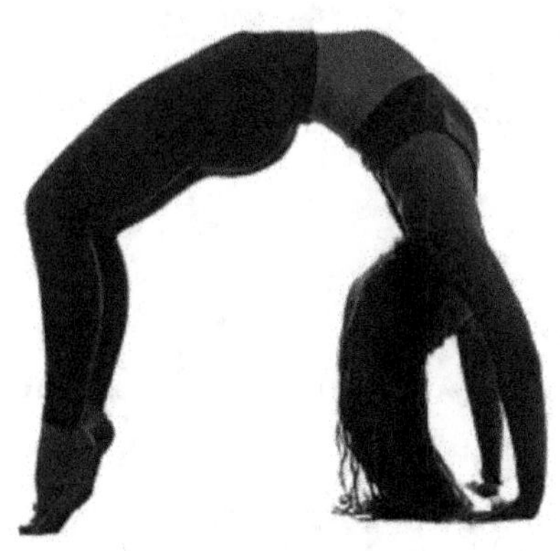

Cat Pose

Category: Beginner

The two simplest and most basic introductory yoga poses **are the cow pose and the cat pose.** They provide an exceptional spinal stretch that can help avoid back pain, keep a good posture, and produce a healthy spine. They **make a**

wonderful addition to a morning or evening activity to allow you to unwind and get ready for bed at night.

Direction

- ✓ Begin on your hands and knees, with your back level, and set like a tabletop pose.

- ✓ Your knees should be just unyouryour hips and your wrists should be immediately beneath your shoulders.

- ✓ Breathe in deeply while bending your back as you sense your abdomen being drawn toward the sky.

✓ Maintain for ten seconds. Relax your back's curve as you breathe out before transitioning into the Cow pose.

✓ Return through the cow, table, and cat positions five times, maintaining each of them for ten seconds.

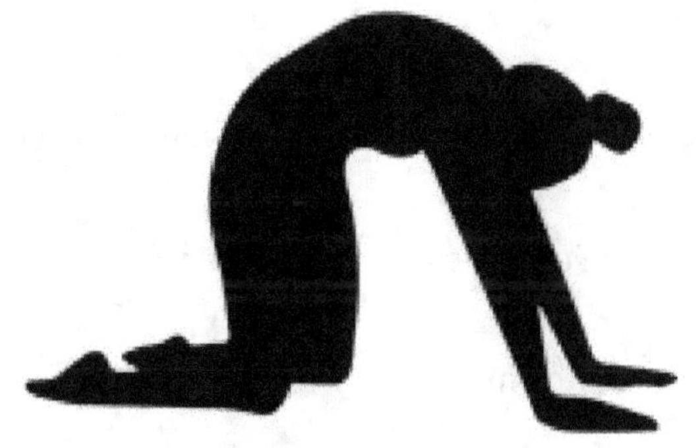

Cow Pose

Category: Beginner

Directions

- ✓ Start on your hands and knees on your yoga mat.

- ✓ Your hands should be shoulder distance apart, slightly in front of your shoulders, and your knees should be beneath your hips.

- ✓ Put your hands down well secured.

- ✓ Raise your chin and chest while lowering your stomach to curve your back and expand your chest as you breathe in.

- ✓ To extend your upper back, concentrate on lengthening the back of your neck and maintaining your abdominal muscles contracted.

✓ Pause between breaths.

✓ Bring your spine to a safe position once you're
prepared to leave the pose.

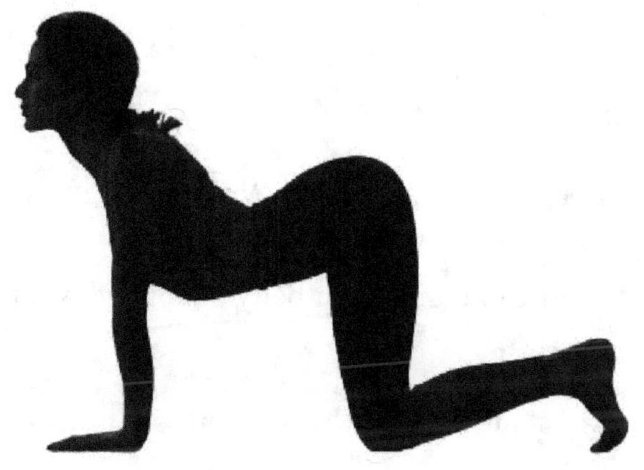

Balancing Table Pose

Category: Beginner

The Balanced Table Pose increases core strength and lower back stiffness. The difficulty of balancing also helps with enhancing concentration, coordination, and general physical proficiency.

Directions

- ✓ Begin in the table pose. Without curving your back, picture dragging your belly button into your spine.

- ✓ Maintain your spine straight and strong as you stretch your right leg behind you.

- ✓ Using your abdominal muscles, extend your left arm forward at shoulder height and level to the floor.

✓ Picture a cord tugging your right leg straight back and your left arm forward while maintaining a straight posture.

✓ Retain for ten seconds then breathe out, and then return to the tabletop pose.

✓ Switch to the other side and repeat the process.

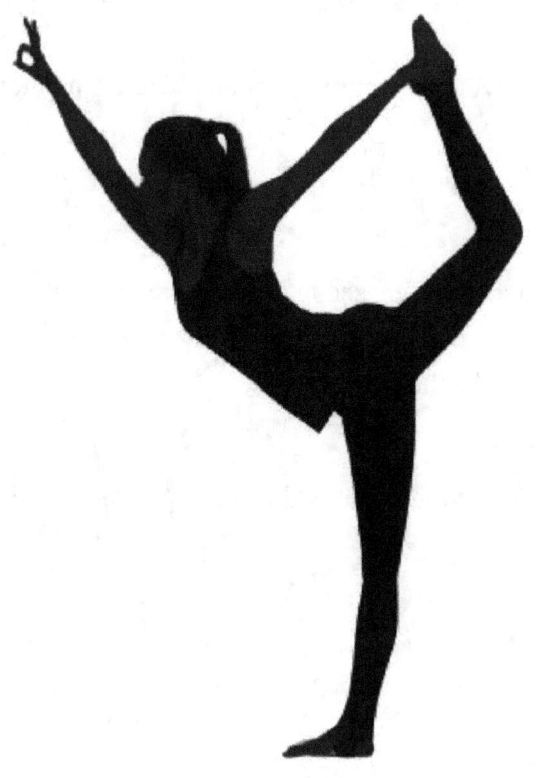

Reverse Tabletop Pose

Category: Beginner

The Reverse Tabletop Pose strengthens the front of the body, the shoulders, the arms, the wrists, and the legs. Also, it enhances posture and offers you a nice energy spike.

Directions

- ✓ To begin, introduce this pose with a staff poses with your legs straight.

- ✓ Curve your knees to place your feet flat on the floor. Provide sufficient room between your feet and your hips so that your knees will meet at a 90-degree angle when you stand up.

✓ Put both hands behind you on the mat, breathe in, and raise your hips while tightly squeezing your hands and feet together.

✓ Stretch your arms, ensure that your knees are at a 90-degree angle, and place your wrist squarely beneath your shoulder with your torso and thigh level with the ground.

✓ Maintain a neutral spine or, if it feels more comfortable, drop your head back. Try to maintain the position by resting your buttocks and using only the weight of your legs.

✓ Maintain the position for between twenty and sixty seconds, then rest back down on the floor.

✓ Do this as much as you can.

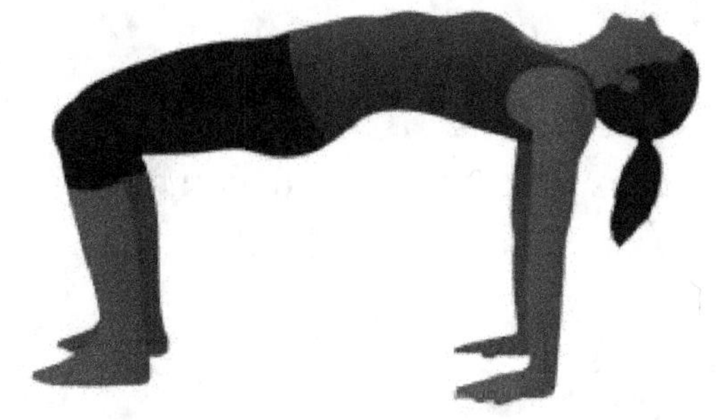

Sphinx Pose

Category: Beginner

Similar to the Cobra Pose, the Sphinx Pose extends the abdominal muscles, tightens the spine, and contracts the buttocks while extending and opening the chest, lungs, and shoulders. However, it balances weight on the forearms rather than the right and gives the spine considerably less curve.

The Sphinx Pose is a tweaked form of the Cobra Pose.

Directions

- ✓ Start by lying face down on your stomach with your legs straight behind you, hip-width spread.

✓ Take a deep breath in and extend your arms straight to the front while pushing your forearms into the ground.

✓ Your shoulders will be raised off the ground by this. Establish a tiny bow in your spine by pushing your shoulders to the back and your pubic bone into the ground.

✓ Maintain this position for ten to twenty seconds, then gradually drop your head, chest, and back to the ground while breathing out.

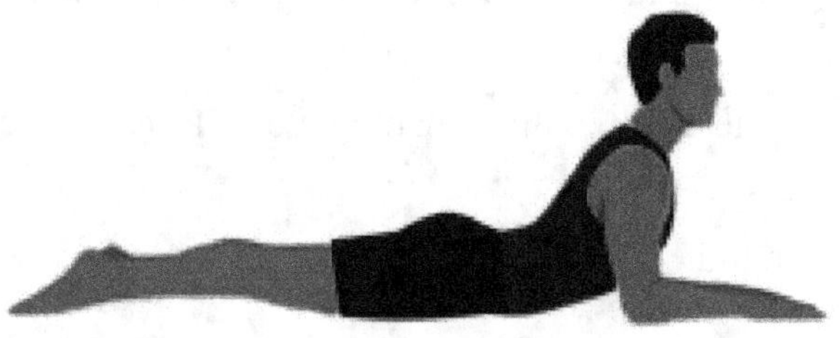

Cobra Pose

Category: Beginner

The Cobra Pose extends the abdominal muscles, enhances the spine, shapes the buttocks, and stretches and opens the chest, lungs, and shoulders.

Directions

- ✓ Begin by laying face-down on the ground with your legs straight behind you, spaced a few inches distant.

✓ Put your hands just underneath your shoulders as if you were getting ready to do a push-up.

✓ Embrace your elbows close to your body and push down on the ground while elevating your torso off the floor but maintaining your lower ribs and pubic bone pushed into the ground.

✓ Just extend your arms to the extent your body would permit. You will be able to fully extend your arms with training; nevertheless should not lock the elbows. Maintain the pose for between thirty and sixty seconds before relaxing back to the ground.

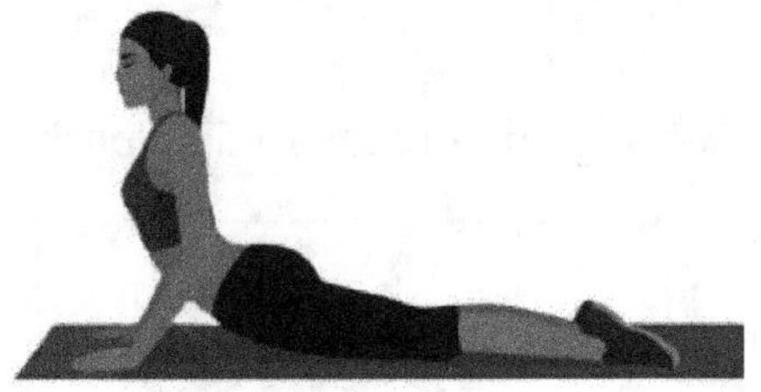

Child's Pose

Category: Beginner

The Child's Pose assists in softly extending the lower back, hips, shoulders, knees, and ankles; calming the spine, shoulders, and neck; and enhancing circulation to the head.

This is just one of the numerous yoga poses that is a fantastic warm-up and a fantastic way to unwind in the night before sleep.

Directions

- ✓ Begin by kneeling with your knees extended nearly as broad as your hips.

- ✓ Breathe out and move to the front until your torso is resting between your thighs and your head is resting on the ground.

- ✓ Put your arms next to your outer thighs with the palms pointing up or stretch them above your head on the floor in front of you.

- ✓ Calm, breathe gradually, and sit down.

- ✓ Gradually straighten your spine while breathing out, diving farther into the pose. Maintain for a three-five

min, breathing gradually and intensifying posture
while breathing.

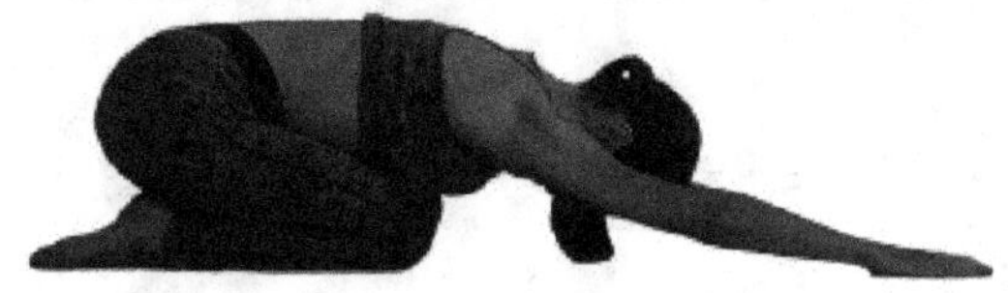

Garland Pose

Category: Beginner

The Garland Pose tones the abdomen while strengthening
the ankles, groin, and back.

Directions

- ✓ Begin by adopting a forward-facing position while keeping your feet hip-width apart. After taking a few long breaths in and out, squat down by lowering your hips.

- ✓ Maintain a straight back and your weight should be on your feet. You can support your heels with a block or cushion if they aren't flat on the ground.

- ✓ Your elbows should be pressed on the inside of your knees as you bring your hands together in front of your chest.

- ✓ Maintain the position for as long as is safe, between five and ten breaths.

✓ Place your hands on the ground, lengthen your legs, and come to a forward bend to exit the position.

✓ Repeat the stance three to five times after pausing for a few breaths.

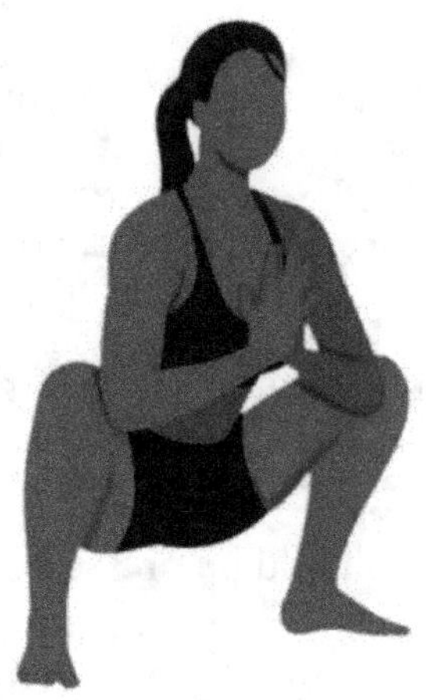

Plank Pose

Category: Beginner

Another popular yoga stance is the "Plank pose," which is frequently appropriated for use in other kinds of fitness challenges. It is a simple pose, yet highly efficient, and can be helpful for both beginner and experienced trainees because the more you keep the pose, the tougher it becomes. The plank pose develops the arms, back, and spine, though it's especially helpful for toning and extending the core.

Directions

- ✓ Ensure your hands and knees are perfectly in line with your shoulders and your hips as you get down on all fours on the ground.

- ✓ Push up through your hands while extending both of your legs behind you so that your body is in a straight line from head to heels.

- ✓ Make sure your body remains in a straight line as you keep it there while engaging your core muscles.

- ✓ To prevent hurting your neck, position your head in line with your body while gazing down at the floor.

- ✓ Maintain the position as much as you can, gradually building up to a minute or more by starting with ten to thirty seconds.

✓ Once you're ready to exit the position, return gradually down to the initial position which is the all four.

✓ Perform the exercise numerous times, taking a thirty-second break between rounds.

✓ To ensure normal form and balance during the workout, keep your breathing steady and contract your core muscles.

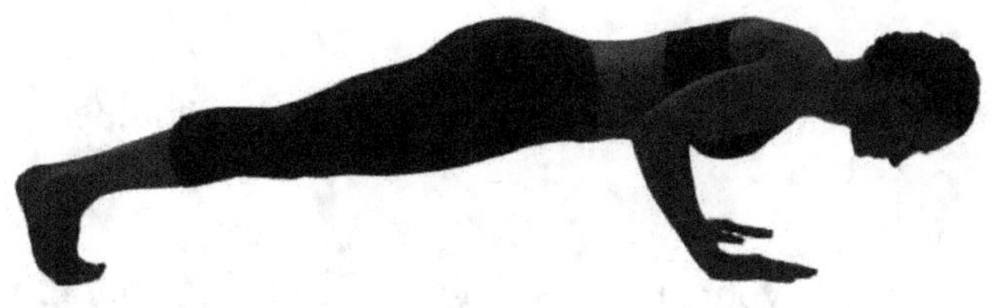

Downward-facing Dog

Category: Beginner

One of the most well-known yoga poses is a downward-facing dog and with valid reason. It is a remarkably adaptable pose that offers an all-around. It also makes a great transition between standing poses and floor postures as well as between different types of floor postures.

Directions

- ✓ Start on your hands and knees with your knees under your hips and your wrists under your shoulders.

- ✓ Extend your arms and legs while raising your hips up and back. Curl your toes beneath.

- ✓ Stretch the crown of your head to the ground while pushing your heels into the ground to extend your spine.

- ✓ Using the muscles in your shoulders and arms, expand your fingers widely and press hard into the palms.

- ✓ Let the gravity of your head drop naturally to the ground while maintaining a calm neck and head.

- ✓ Maintain this position for between thirty and sixty seconds while breathing in deeply and breathing out to relieve any muscle pain.

✓ Flex your knees and lower them to the ground again

to exit the downward dog position.

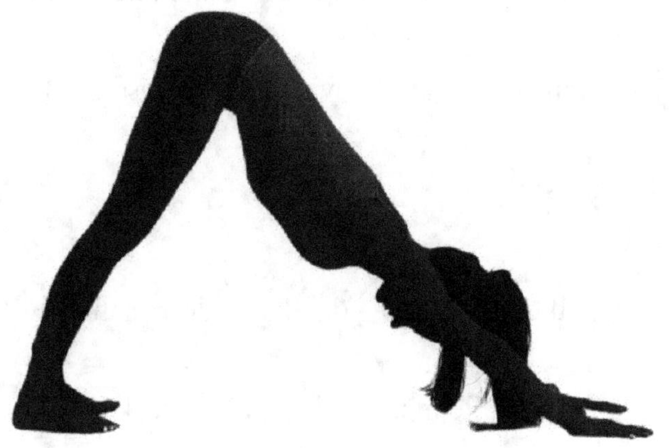

Upward-facing Dog

Category: Beginner

Upward-facing Dog Pose improves the spine, shapes the buttocks, and extends the abdominal muscles while expanding and opening the chest, lungs, and shoulders.

Directions

- ✓ Start by laying face down on the ground with your arms by your side and your hands beneath your shoulders.

- ✓ Raising your chest off the floor, solidly pressing your hands into the ground, straightening your arms.

✓ Maintain a straight posture while planting the tops of

your feet firmly on the floor.

✓ Lift your thighs off the floor by contracting the

muscles in your core.

✓ Stretching your neck and lining it up with your spine,

raise your eyes upward.

✓ After a few seconds, keep the position before

releasing it onto the ground again.

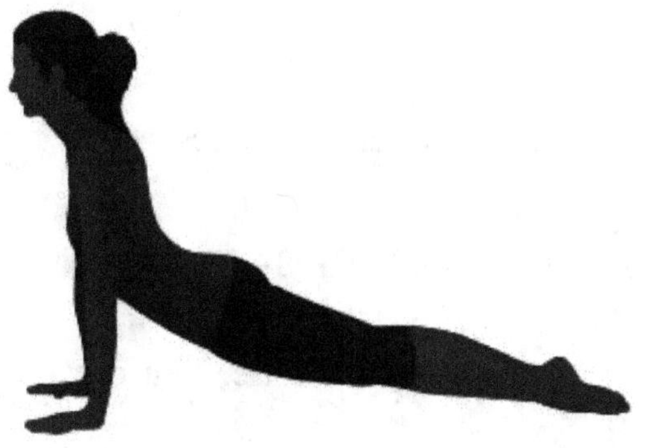

CONCLUSION

Beginner yoga classes, which are created especially for those with little or little previous knowledge, are where you should start if you're a novice to the exercise. You can gradually develop your strength and flexibility while learning the fundamental poses.

Having a competent teacher is vital for any type of learning, and it's no different in the case of yoga. A skilled trainer can show you the proper poses, breathing techniques, and meditations.

Yoga is a comprehensive activity that addresses one's bodily, psychological, and emotional health; it's not a form of game.

Which is why, rather than speeding through to the postures to catch pace with the others, concentrate on your technique, maintain your calmness, and then intimate with the process.

Yoga needs consistent practice in order to provide the intended outcomes. Include it in your daily schedule, even if it's just for some minutes, and as your training improves, gradually extend the duration.

Pay attention to your body's cues and don't strain yourself too far. Reverse a stance if it causes you pain or discomfort and adjusts it to your demands.

Yoga is about maintaining a healthy way of life as well as physical practice. Thus, watch what you eat, have a balanced diet, and drink enough water prior to and after the activity.

Finally, have fun on the way. Yoga is a lifetime habit that has enormous advantages for your bodily, psychological, and emotional health. Hence, take pleasure in the procedure, accept the difficulties and benefit from it.